52 Weight Gaining Shake Recipes to Get Bigger Faster:

Naturally Increase in Size In 4 Weeks or Less!

By

Joe Correa CSN

COPYRIGHT

© 2017 Live Stronger Faster Inc.

This publication is designed to provide accurate and authoritative information in regard to the subject matter covered. It is sold with the understanding that neither the author nor the publisher is engaged in rendering medical advice. If medical advice or assistance is needed, consult with a doctor. This book is considered a guide and should not be used in any way detrimental to your health. Consult with a physician before starting this nutritional plan to make sure it's right for you.

ACKNOWLEDGEMENTS

This book is dedicated to my friends and family that have had mild or serious illnesses so that you may find a solution and make the necessary changes in your life.

52 Weight Gaining Shake Recipes to Get Bigger Faster:

Naturally Increase in Size In 4 Weeks or Less!

By

Joe Correa CSN

CONTENTS

Copyright

Acknowledgements

About The Author

Introduction

52 Weight Gaining Shake Recipes to Get Bigger Faster: Naturally Increase in Size In 4 Weeks or Less!

Additional Titles from This Author

ABOUT THE AUTHOR

After years of Research, I honestly believe in the positive effects that proper nutrition can have over the body and mind. My knowledge and experience has helped me live healthier throughout the years and which I have shared with family and friends. The more you know about eating and drinking healthier, the sooner you will want to change your life and eating habits.

Nutrition is a key part in the process of being healthy and living longer so get started today. The first step is the most important and the most significant.

INTRODUCTION

52 Weight Gaining Shake Recipes to Get Bigger Faster: Naturally Increase in Size In 4 Weeks or Less!

By Joe Correa CSN

Fighting to gain weight can be difficult for many people who have a fast metabolism. The key is to gain weight in a healthy manner so you can manage your weight.

Being too heavy or too thin are unhealthy extremes. Although you want to eat foods with additional calories, gaining extra pounds is not that simple. First of all, you need 5 to 6 meals a day and eat smaller portions. This can take some time to making it your new normal way of eating.

An easy and healthy way to add calories is by supplementing some meals with weight gaining juices or shakes. You have to learn to trick your body into taking more calories than usual and the best way to do it lies in a juicer. Juicing different ingredients and ingesting highly nutritious foods will provide your body with some weight gaining benefits:

1. Your body will skip the usual mechanism of chewing food and feeling satisfied within a short period of time

2. Juice is not a meal! Or at least that's what we are taught. This is partly true – juicing doesn't include the typical solid meal we're used to. A proper juice recipe, on the other hand, will provide more than enough nutrients to help you gain some healthy weight.
3. A healthy juice recipe will speed up your metabolism which will result in an increased need for food.
4. Calories you consume in a healthy juice recipe will help improve your overall health.

Never replace your meals with juices or shakes. Bear in mind that a balanced diet combined with healthy juices is the best way to gain weight.

This collection of juice recipes contains carefully chosen juices that are based on healthy and high-calorie foods. These juices are easy to make and are loaded with different nutrients your body needs to build muscle.

52 WEIGHT GAINING SHAKE RECIPES TO GET BIGGER FASTER: NATURALLY INCREASE IN SIZE IN 4 WEEKS OR LESS!

1.   Celery Apple Juice

Ingredients:

1 large green apple, cored

1 large lemon, peeled

3 large celery stalks, chopped

1 large cucumber

2 oz of coconut water

Preparation:

Wash the apple and cut lengthwise in half. Remove the core and cut into small chunks. Set aside.

Peel the lemon and cut lengthwise in half. Set aside.

Wash the celery stalks and cut into small pieces. Set aside.

Peel the cucumber and cut into small chunks. Set aside.

Now, combine apple, lemon, celery, and cucumber in a juicer and process until well juiced. Transfer to serving glasses and stir in the coconut water.

Add few ice cubes and serve immediately.

Enjoy!

Nutritional information per serving: Kcal: 175, Protein: 5.1g, Carbs: 50.2g, Fats: 1.3g

2.   Mixed Berry Juice

Ingredients:

1 cup of blackberries

1 cup of blueberries

3 large strawberries, chopped

1 large lime, peeled

1 large cucumber, chopped

1 cup of fresh mint, torn

2 oz of water

Preparation:

Combine blackberries and blueberries in a colander. Rinse under cold running water and drain. Set aside.

Wash the strawberries and remove the stems, if any. Cut into bite-sized pieces and set aside.

Peel the lime and cut lengthwise in half. Set aside.

Wash the cucumber and cut into small chunks. Set aside.

Wash the mint and torn with hands. Set aside.

Now, combine blackberries, blueberries, strawberries, cucumber, and mint in a juicer and process until juiced. Transfer to serving glasses and stir in the water.

Add some ice or refrigerate for 15 minutes before serving.

Nutritional information per serving: Kcal: 173, Protein: 6.6g, Carbs: 57.8g, Fats: 1.9g

3.   Cherry Banana Juice

Ingredients:

2 cups of cherries, pitted

1 large banana, chunked

1 large lime, peeled

2 large green apples, chopped

¼ tsp of cinnamon

1 oz of water

Preparation:

Rinse the cherries under cold running water and drain. Cut each in half and remove the pits. Set aside.

Peel the banana and chop into chunks. Set aside.

Peel the lime and cut lengthwise in half. Set aside.

Wash the apples and cut lengthwise in half. Remove the core and cut into small chunks.

Now, combine cherries, banana, lime, and apples in a juicer and process until well juiced.

Transfer to a serving glass and stir in the cinnamon and water. Add some ice before serving and enjoy!

Nutritional information per serving: Kcal: 297, Protein: 4.2g, Carbs: 87.5g, Fats: 1.2g

4.   Raspberry Carrot Juice

Ingredients:

1 cup of raspberries

2 large carrots, peeled and chopped

1 large orange, wedged

¼ tsp of ginger, ground

1 tbsp of liquid honey

Preparation:

Using a colander, rinse the raspberries under cold running water and drain. Set aside.

Wash the carrots and peel them. Cut into small chunks and set aside.

Peel the orange and divide into wedges. Set aside.

Now, combine raspberries, carrots, and orange in a juicer and process until well juiced. Transfer to a serving glass and stir in the ginger and honey.

Refrigerate for 15 minutes before serving.

Nutritional information per serving: Kcal: 204, Protein: 4.5g, Carbs: 67.1g, Fats: 1.3g

5.   Apricot Orange Juice

Ingredients:

2 whole apricots, pitted

1 large orange, wedged

1 cup of green grapes

1 small ginger slice, peeled

1 oz of water

Preparation:

Wash the apricots and cut lengthwise in half. Remove the pits and cut into bite-sized pieces. Set aside.

Peel the orange and divide into wedges. Set aside.

Wash the grapes and set aside.

Peel the ginger slice and cut into small pieces. Set aside.

Now, combine apricots, orange, grapes, and ginger in a juicer. Process until juiced and transfer to a serving glass. Add some ice before serving.

Enjoy!

Nutritional information per serving: Kcal: 157, Protein: 3.3g, Carbs: 45.7g, Fats: 0.8g

6.   Cauliflower Basil Juice

Ingredients:

1 cup of cauliflower, chopped

1 cup of fresh basil, torn

1 cup of broccoli, chopped

1 cup of beet greens, torn

1 large lemon, peeled

1 medium-sized red apple, cored

Preparation:

Trim off the outer leaves of a cauliflower. Wash it and fill and cut into small pieces. Fill the measuring cup and reserve the rest in the refrigerator.

Combine basil and beet greens in a large colander. Rinse under cold running water and drain. Torn with hands and set aside.

Wash the broccoli and chop into small pieces. Set aside.

Peel the lemon and cut lengthwise in half. Set aside.

Wash the apple and cut lengthwise in half. Remove the core and cut into bite-sized pieces. Set aside.

Now, combine cauliflower, basil, broccoli, beet greens, lemon, and apple in a juicer. Process until well juiced and transfer to a serving glass.

Add few ice cubes and serve immediately.

Nutritional information per serving: Kcal: 137, Protein: 7.3g, Carbs: 42.1g, Fats: 1.3g

7.   Ginger Artichoke Juice

Ingredients:

1 medium-sized artichoke, chopped

1 small ginger slice, peeled

3 medium-sized celery stalks

2 large kiwis, peeled

1 tbsp of liquid honey

Preparation:

Trim off the outer leaves of the artichoke using a sharp paring knife. Wash it and cut into bite-sized pieces. Set aside.

Peel the ginger slice and cut into small pieces. Set aside.

Wash the celery stalks and cut into bite-sized pieces. Set aside.

Peel the kiwis and cut lengthwise in half. Set aside.

Now, combine artichoke, ginger, celery, and kiwi in a juicer. Process until well juiced and transfer to a serving glass. Stir in the honey and refrigerate for 15 minutes before serving.

Enjoy!

Nutritional information per serving: Kcal: 174, Protein: 6.6g, Carbs: 54.6g, Fats: 1.2g

8.   Guava Mango Juice

Ingredients:

1 large guava, chopped

1 cup of mango, chunked

1 medium-sized banana, chopped

1 large orange, wedged

1 oz of coconut water

Preparation:

Wash and peel the guava and mango. Cut into small chunks and set aside.

Peel the banana and cut into small chunks. Set aside.

Peel the orange and divide into wedges. Set aside.

Now, combine guava, mango, banana, and orange in a juicer and process until well juiced. Transfer to a serving glass and stir in the water.

Add some ice and serve immediately.

Enjoy!

Nutritional information per serving: Kcal: 275, Protein: 5.7g, Carbs: 81.1g, Fats: 1.8g

9.　　Avocado Mango Juice

Ingredients:

1 cup of avocado, cubed

1 medium-sized mango

1large orange, wedged

¼ tsp of ginger, ground

3 tbsp of coconut water

Preparation:

Peel the avocado and cut lengthwise in half. Remove the pit and cut into small cubes. Fill the measuring cup and reserve the rest to a refrigerator.

Peel the mango and cut into small chunks. Set aside.

Peel the orange and divide into wedges. Cut each wedge in half and set aside.

Now, combine avocado, mango, and orange in a juicer and process until well juiced. Transfer to a serving glass and stir in the ginger and coconut water.

Add some ice and serve immediately.

Nutritional information per serving: Kcal: 457, Protein: 8.1g, Carbs: 84.7g, Fats: 23.5g

10.   Apple Carrot Juice

Ingredients:

1 medium-sized apple, cored

1 medium-sized carrot, chopped

1 whole lemon, peeled

1 large peach, pitted

2 oz of water

¼ tsp of cinnamon, ground

Preparation:

Wash the apple and cut lengthwise in half. Remove the core and cut into bite-sized pieces. Set aside.

Wash and peel the carrot. Cut into small chunks and set aside.

Peel the lemon and cut lengthwise in half. Set aside.

Wash the peach and cut in half. Remove the pit and cut into bite-sized pieces. Set aside.

Now, combine apple, carrot, lemon, and peach in a juicer. Process until nicely juiced. Transfer to a serving glass and stir in the water and cinnamon.

Add some ice or refrigerate for 10 minutes before serving.

Enjoy!

Nutritional information per serving: Kcal: 165, Protein: 3.6g, Carbs: 50.7g, Fats: 1.1g

11. Beet Lemon Juice

Ingredients:

2 large beets, trimmed and chopped

1 whole lemon, peeled

1 cup of broccoli, chopped

1 large cucumber, sliced

Preparation:

Wash the beets and trim off the green parts. Cut into bite-sized pieces and set aside.

Peel the lemon and cut lengthwise in half. Set aside.

Wash the broccoli and cut into bite-sized pieces. Fill the measuring cup and reserve the rest for later.

Wash the cucumber and cut into thin slices. Set aside.

Now, combine beets, lemon, broccoli, and cucumber in a juicer and process until juiced. Transfer to a serving glass and add some ice before serving.

Enjoy!

Nutritional information per serving: Kcal: 123, Protein: 7.8g, Carbs: 38.1g, Fats: 1.1g

12.   Fennel Collard Green Juice

Ingredients:

1 cup of fennel, chopped

1 cup of collard greens, torn

1 large leek, chopped

1 cup of fresh mint, torn

1 large green apple, cored

A handful of spinach

1 tbsp of liquid honey

Preparation:

Wash the fennel bulb and trim off the wilted outer layers. Cut into small chunks and fill the measuring cup. Reserve the rest in the refrigerator.

In a large colander, combine collard greens, mint, and spinach. Rinse thoroughly under cold running water and drain. Torn with hands and set aside.

Wash the leek and cut into bite-sized pieces. Set aside.

Wash the apple and cut in half. Remove the core and cut into bite-sized pieces. Set aside.

Now, combine fennel, collard greens, mint, spinach, leek, and apple in a juicer. Process until well juiced.

Transfer to a serving glass and refrigerate for 15 minutes before serving.

Nutritional information per serving: Kcal: 180, Protein: 6.2g, Carbs: 53.7g, Fats: 1.4g

13.   Blueberry Banana Juice

Ingredients:

1 cup of blueberries

1 medium-sized banana, chopped

1 whole lime, peeled

1 large pear, chopped

1 cup of blackberries

1 large orange, wedged

Preparation:

In a large colander, combine blueberries and blackberries. Rinse well under cold running water and drain. Set aside.

Peel the banana and chop into chunks. Set aside.

Peel the lime and cut lengthwise in half. Set aside.

Wash the pear and cut in half. Remove the core and cut into bite-sized pieces. Set aside.

Peel the orange and divide into wedges. Set aside.

Now, combine blueberries, blackberries, banana, lime, pear, and orange in a juicer and process until well juiced.

Transfer to a serving glass and add some crushed ice.

Enjoy!

Nutritional information per serving: Kcal: 376, Protein: 7.2g, Carbs: 122.6g, Fats: 2.6g

14.   Pineapple Orange Juice

Ingredients:

1 cup of pineapple chunks

1 medium-sized orange, peeled

1 small carrot, chopped

1 whole lime, peeled

1 tbsp of liquid honey

Preparation:

Cut the top of a pineapple and peel it using a sharp knife. Cut into small chunks. Reserve the rest of the pineapple in a refrigerator.

Peel the orange and divide into wedges. Cut each wedge in half and set aside.

Peel the carrot and cut into thin slices. Set aside.

Peel the lime and cut lengthwise in half. Set aside.

Now, combine pineapple, orange, carrot, and lime in a juicer and process until well juiced. Transfer to a serving glass and stir in the honey.

Refrigerate for 15 minutes before serving.

Nutritional information per serving: Kcal: 207, Protein: 2.7g, Carbs: 61.5g, Fats: 0.7g

15. Peach Plum Juice

Ingredients:

2 medium-sized peaches, pitted

2 whole plums, pitted

1 whole lemon, peeled

1 cup of watermelon

¼ tsp of ginger, ground

Preparation:

Wash the peaches and cut in half. Remove the pits and cut into bite-sized pieces. Set aside.

Wash the plums and cut lengthwise in half. Remove the pits and set aside.

Peel the lemons and cut lengthwise in half. Set aside.

Cut the watermelon lengthwise. For one cup, you will need a large slice. Peel and cut into chunks. Remove the seeds and set aside. Reserve the rest for some other juices.

Now, combine peaches, plums, lemon, and watermelon in a juicer and process until juiced. Transfer to a serving glass and stir in the ginger.

Refrigerate for 10 minutes before serving.

Nutritional information per serving: Kcal: 205, Protein: 5.2g, Carbs: 60.6g, Fats: 1.5g

16. Red Pepper Tomato Juice

Ingredients:

2 large red bell peppers, chopped

3 cherry tomatoes, halved

1 cup of fresh parsley, chopped

1 medium-sized carrot, sliced

1 tsp of fresh rosemary, finely chopped

Preparation:

Wash the bell peppers and cut lengthwise in half. Remove the seeds and cut into small pieces. Set aside.

Wash the tomatoes and cut in half. Set aside.

Rinse the parsley under cold running water and chop into small pieces.

Wash and peel the carrot. Cut into thin slices and set aside.

Now, combine bell peppers, tomatoes, parsley, carrot, and rosemary in a juicer and process until juiced.

Transfer to a serving glass and refrigerate for 10 minutes before serving.

Nutritional information per serving: Kcal: 112, Protein: 6.1g, Carbs: 31.4g, Fats: 1.7g

17.   Squash Kiwi Juice

Ingredients:

1 cup of crookneck squash

1 whole kiwi, peeled

1 medium-sized orange, peeled

1 cup of fresh kale, torn

1 tbsp of liquid honey

1 oz of water

Preparation:

Peel the crookneck squash and scrape out the seeds with a spoon. Cut into small cubes and fill the measuring cup. Reserve the rest of the squash for some other recipe. Wrap in a plastic foil and refrigerate.

Peel the kiwi and cut lengthwise in half. Set aside.

Peel the orange and divide into wedges. Set aside.

Rinse the kale under cold running water and slightly drain. Torn with hands and set aside.

Now, combine crookneck squash, kiwi, orange, and kale in a juicer. Process until well juiced and transfer to a serving glass.

Stir in the honey and water. Add some ice before serving and enjoy!

Nutritional information per serving: Kcal: 126, Protein: 6.2g, Carbs: 36.3g, Fats: 1.5g

18. Asparagus Avocado Juice

Ingredients:

1 cup of fresh asparagus, trimmed

1 cup of avocado, cubed

1 whole lime, peeled

1 cup of Swiss chard, torn

1 small Golden Delicious apple, cored

1 small ginger knob, peeled

Preparation:

Wash the asparagus and trim off the woody ends. Cut into bite-sized pieces and set aside.

Peel the avocado and cut lengthwise in half. Remove the pit and cut into small chunks. Set aside.

Peel the lime and cut lengthwise in half. Set aside.

Rinse the Swiss chard thoroughly under cold running water and slightly drain. Torn with hands and set aside.

Peel the ginger knob and cut into small pieces. Set aside.

Now, process asparagus, avocado, lime, chard, and ginger in a juicer. Transfer to a serving glass and refrigerate for 15 minutes before serving.

Enjoy!

Nutritional information per serving: Kcal: 298, Protein: 7.3g, Carbs: 41.6g, Fats: 22.5g

19.   Artichoke Tomato Juice

Ingredients:

1 medium-sized artichoke, chopped

1 medium-sized tomato, chopped

1 medium-sized bell pepper, chopped

1 garlic clove, peeled

1 cup of cucumber, sliced

1 tsp of balsamic vinegar

¼ tsp of salt

Preparation:

Using a sharp knife, trim off the outer leaves of the artichoke. Wash it and cut into bite-sized pieces. Set aside.

Wash the tomato and place it in a small bowl. Cut into small pieces, but make sure to keep the juices while cutting. Set aside.

Wash the pepper and cut in half. Remove the seeds and chop into small pieces. Set aside.

Wash the cucumber and cut into thin slices. Fill the measuring cup and refrigerate the rest for later.

Now, combine artichoke, tomato, bell pepper, garlic, and cucumber in a juicer and process until juiced.

Transfer to a serving glass and stir in the vinegar and salt. You can sprinkle with some fresh rosemary for some extra taste. However, it is optional.

Refrigerate for 10 minutes before serving.

Nutritional information per serving: Kcal: 86, Protein: 7g, Carbs: 28.3g, Fats: 0.9g

20.   Brussels Sprouts Juice

Ingredients:

2 cups of Brussels sprouts, halved

1 medium-sized Granny Smith's apple, cored

1 cup of fresh mint, torn

1 cup of fresh kale, torn

1 whole lime, peeled

1 oz of water

Preparation:

Wash the Brussels sprouts and trim off the outer leaves. Cut in half and fill the measuring cup. Reserve the rest for later.

Wash the apple and cut in half. Remove the core and cut into bite-sized pieces. Set aside.

Combine mint and kale in a large colander and rinse under cold running water. Slightly drain and torn with hands. Set aside.

Peel the lime and cut lengthwise in half. Set aside.

Now, combine Brussels sprouts, apple, mint, kale, and lime in a juicer and process until juiced. Transfer to a serving glass and stir in the water.

Refrigerate for 10 minutes before serving.

Enjoy!

Nutritional information per serving: Kcal: 171, Protein: 10.6g, Carbs: 51.7g, Fats: 1.7g

21.   Parsnip Carrot Juice

Ingredients:

2 cups of parsnip, sliced

1 medium-sized carrot, sliced

1 cup of cucumber, sliced

1 cup of watercress, torn

1 whole lemon, peeled

1 small ginger knob, peeled

Preparation:

Wash and peel the parsnip and carrot. Cut into thin slices and set aside.

Peel the cucumber and chop into chunks. Fill the measuring cup and reserve the rest for later.

Rinse the watercress under cold running water and slightly drain. Torn with hands and set aside.

Peel the lemon and cut lengthwise in half. Set aside.

Peel the ginger knob and cut into small pieces. Set aside.

Now, combine parsnip, carrot, cucumber, watercress, lemon, and ginger in a juicer and process until well juiced.

Transfer to a serving glass and add few ice cubes before serving.

Nutritional information per serving: Kcal: 192, Protein: 5.6g, Carbs: 62.5g, Fats: 1.3g

22.   Cauliflower Broccoli Juice

Ingredients:

1 cup of cauliflower, chopped

1 cup of broccoli, chopped

1 small green apple, cored

1 cup of fresh kale, torn

¼ teaspoon of ginger, ground

Preparation:

Wash the cauliflower and trim off the outer leaves. Cut into small pieces and set aside.

Wash the broccoli thoroughly and chop into small pieces. Set aside.

Wash the apple and cut lengthwise in half. remove the core and cut into bite-sized pieces. Set aside.

Rinse the kale under cold running water and slightly drain. Torn with hands and set aside.

Now, combine cauliflower, broccoli, apple, and kale in a juicer and process until well juiced. Transfer to a serving glass and stir in the ground ginger.

Refrigerate for 20 minutes before serving.

Nutritional information per serving: Kcal: 131, Protein: 8.1g, Carbs: 36.8g, Fats: 1.5g

23. Blackberry Lemon Juice

Ingredients:

1 cup of blackberries

1 whole lemon, peeled

1 cup of cucumber, sliced

1 cup of beets, sliced

1 oz of coconut water

Preparation:

Using a small colander, rinse the blackberries under cold running water. Slightly drain and set aside.

Peel the lemon and cut lengthwise in half. Set aside.

Wash the cucumber and cut into thin slices. Fill the measuring cup and reserve the rest in the refrigerator for some other juice.

Wash the beets and trim off the green parts. Cut into bite-sized pieces and fill the measuring cup. Reserve the rest for later.

Now, combine blackberries, lemon, cucumber, and beets in a juicer and process until juiced. Transfer to a serving glass and stir in the coconut water. Add some ice and serve immediately.

Nutritional information per serving: Kcal: 103, Protein: 5.2g, Carbs: 34.2g, Fats: 1.2g

24.   Fennel Asparagus Juice

Ingredients:

1 cup of fennel, chopped

1 cup of asparagus, trimmed and chopped

1 cup of avocado, sliced

2 medium-sized carrots

1 tbsp of liquid honey

Preparation:

Wash the fennel bulb and trim off the wilted outer layers. Cut into small chunks and fill the measuring cup. Reserve the rest for some other juice.

Wash the asparagus and trim off the woody ends. Cut into bite-sized pieces and fill the measuring cup. Refrigerate the rest for later.

Peel the avocado and cut lengthwise in half. Remove the pit and cut into thin slices. Fill the measuring cup and reserve the rest for later.

Wash and peel the carrots. Cut into small chunks and set aside.

Now, combine fennel, asparagus, avocado, and carrots in a juicer and process until well juiced. Transfer to a serving glass and stir in the honey.

Refrigerate for 15 minutes before serving.

Nutritional information per serving: Kcal: 263, Protein: 8.1g, Carbs: 35.7g, Fats: 22.1g

25.   Cantaloupe Mango Juice

Ingredients:

1 cup of cantaloupe, diced

1 cup of mango, chunked

1 medium-sized peach, pitted

1 whole lime, peeled

1 cup of fresh mint, finely chopped

Preparation:

Cut the cantaloupe in half. Scoop out the seeds and cut two wedges and peel them. Chop into chunks and set aside. Reserve the rest of the cantaloupe in a refrigerator.

Wash and peel the mango. Cut into small chunks and set aside.

Wash the peach and cut lengthwise in half. Remove the pit and cut into bite-sized pieces. Set aside.

Peel the lime and cut lengthwise in half. Set aside.

Now, combine cantaloupe, mango, peach, lime, and mint in a juicer. Process until well juiced. Transfer to a serving glass and add some crushed ice.

Serve immediately.

Nutritional information per serving: Kcal: 205, Protein: 5.2g, Carbs: 59.2g, Fats: 1.6g

26. Pepper Tomato Juice

Ingredients:

1 large red bell pepper, chopped

4 cherry tomatoes, halved

1 small celery stalk, chopped

1 medium-sized radish, chopped

1 small red apple, cored

¼ tsp of cayenne pepper

Preparation:

Wash the bell pepper and cut lengthwise in half. Remove the seeds and cut into small pieces. Set aside.

Wash the cherry tomatoes and place in a small bowl. Cut in half and reserve the tomato juice while cutting.

Wash the celery stalk and cut into small pieces. Set aside.

Wash the radish and trim off the green parts. Slightly peel and cut into small pieces. Set aside.

Wash the apple and cut in half. Remove the core and cut into bite-sized pieces.

Now, combine pepper, tomatoes, celery, radish, and apple in a juicer and process until well juiced. Transfer to serving glass and stir in the cayenne pepper. You can add a pinch of salt, but it's optional.

Refrigerate for 10 minutes before serving.

Nutritional information per serving: Kcal: 129, Protein: 2.9g, Carbs: 35.9g, Fats: 2.9g

27. Avocado Cherry Juice

Ingredients:

1 cup of avocado, cubed

1 cup of fresh cherries, pitted

1 whole lime, peeled

1 medium-sized orange, wedged

1 tbsp of honey, raw

Preparation:

Peel the avocado and cut in half. Remove the pit and cut into small cubes. Fill the measuring cup and reserve the rest for later.

Wash the cherries and cut each in half. Remove the pits and set aside.

Peel the lime and cut lengthwise in half. Set aside.

Peel the orange and divide into wedges. Cut each wedge in half and set aside.

Now, combine avocado, cherries, lime, and orange in a juicer and process until well juiced. Transfer to a serving glass and stir in the honey.

Add some crushed ice and serve.

Nutritional information per serving: Kcal: 408, Protein: 6g, Carbs: 74.5g, Fats: 22.5g

28.   Raspberry Apricot Juice

Ingredients:

1 cup of raspberries

1 cup of apricots, sliced

1 medium-sized carrot, sliced

2 whole plums, pitted

1 tbsp of honey, raw

Preparation:

Using a colander, wash the raspberries in under cold running water. Slightly drain and set aside.

Wash the apricots and cut lengthwise in half. Remove the pits and cut into thin slices. Fill the measuring cup and reserve the rest for later.

Wash and peel the carrot. Cut into thin slices and set aside.

Wash the plums and cut in half. Remove the pits and set aside.

Now, combine raspberries, apricots, carrot, and plums in a juicer and process until well juiced.

Transfer to a serving glass and stir in the honey. Add some crushed ice before serving.

Nutritional information per serving: Kcal: 232, Protein: 5.3g, Carbs: 70.9g, Fats: 1.9g

29.   Beet Kiwi Juice

Ingredients:

1 cup of beets, sliced

1 whole kiwi, sliced

1 small apple, cored

1 small pear, cored

¼ tsp of cinnamon, ground

Preparation:

Wash the beets and trim off the green ends. Peel and cut into thin slices. Fill the measuring cup and reserve the rest for some other juice.

Peel the kiwi and cut lengthwise in half. Set aside.

Wash the apple and pear. Remove the core and cut into bite-sized pieces. Set aside.

Now, combine beets, kiwi, apple, and pear in a juicer and process until well juiced. Transfer to a serving glass and stir in the cinnamon. Refrigerate for 15 minutes before serving.

Enjoy!

Nutritional information per serving: Kcal: 211, Protein: 4.2g, Carbs: 65.3g, Fats: 1.1g

30.   Strawberry Avocado Juice

Ingredients:

1 cup of strawberries, chopped

1 cup of avocado, cubed

1 pomegranate seeds

1 cup of cucumber, sliced

1 medium-sized orange, wedged

Preparation:

Wash the strawberries and cut into small pieces. Set aside.

Peel the avocado and cut in half. Remove the pit and cut into cubes. Fill the measuring cup and reserve the rest for later.

Cut the top of the pomegranate fruit using a sharp paring knife. Slice down to each of the white membranes inside of the fruit. Pop the seeds into a measuring cup and set aside.

Wash the cucumber and cut into thin slices. Fill the measuring cup and reserve the rest for later.

Peel the orange and divide into wedges. Chop each wedge in half and set aside.

Now, combine strawberries, avocado, pomegranate, cucumber, and orange in a juicer. Process until well juiced.

Transfer to a serving glass and add some crushed ice before serving.

Nutritional information per serving: Kcal: 335, Protein: 6.6g, Carbs: 53.2g, Fats: 23.5g

31.   Cherry Mango Juice

Ingredients:

1 cup of fresh cherries

1 cup of mango, chunked

1 cup of fresh mint, torn

1 small apple, cored

¼ tsp of ginger, ground

Preparation:

Wash the cherries and cut each in half. Remove the pits and fill the measuring cup. Reserve the rest for some other juice.

Peel the mango and cut into small chunks. Fill the measuring cup and refrigerate the rest for later.

Wash the mint thoroughly under cold running water. Slightly drain and torn with hands. Set aside.

Wash the apple and cut in half. Remove the core and cut into bite-sized pieces. Set aside.

Now, combine cherries, mango, mint, and apple in a juicer and process until juiced. Transfer to a serving glass and stir in the ginger.

Add some ice or refrigerate for 15 minutes before serving.

Nutritional information per serving: Kcal: 262, Protein: 4.3g, Carbs: 75.3g, Fats: 6.6g

32. Watermelon Grape Juice

Ingredients:

1 cup of watermelon, cubed

1 cup of green grapes

1 whole kiwi, peeled

1 medium-sized pear, chopped

Preparation:

Cut the watermelon lengthwise. Cut one large wedge and peel it. Cut into chunks and fill the measuring cup. Remove the seeds and set aside. Reserve the rest of the melon for some other juices.

Wash the grapes and set aside.

Peel the kiwi and cut lengthwise in half. Set aside.

Wash the pear and remove the core. Cut into bite-sized pieces and set aside.

Now, combine watermelon, grapes, kiwi, and pear in a juicer and process until well juiced.

Transfer to a serving glass and add some crushed ice before serving.

Enjoy!

Nutritional information per serving: Kcal: 216, Protein: 3g, Carbs: 64.5g, Fats: 1.2g

33.   Spinach Kale Juice

Ingredients:

1 cup of fresh spinach, torn

1 cup of fresh kale, torn

1 cup of cabbage, shredded

1 cup of fresh parsley, torn

1 cup of cucumber, sliced

1 cup of avocado, chunked

¼ tsp of turmeric, ground

Preparation:

Combine spinach, kale, and parsley in a large colander. Rinse all under cold running water and slightly drain. Torn with hands and set aside.

Wash the cabbage thoroughly and shred the cabbage. Fill the measuring cup and reserve the rest for later.

Wash the cucumber and cut into thin slices. Set aside.

Peel the avocado and cut in half. Remove the pit and cut into small chunks. Fill the measuring cup and reserve the rest for later.

Now, combine spinach, kale, parsley, cabbage, cucumber, and avocado in a juicer and process until juiced. Transfer to a serving glass and stir in the turmeric.

Refrigerate for 10 minutes and serve.

Nutritional information per serving: Kcal: 272, Protein: 10.9g, Carbs: 33.1g, Fats: 23.5g

34.   Collard Greens Tomato Juice

Ingredients:

1 cup of collard greens, roughly chopped

1 cup of Romaine lettuce, roughly chopped

1 large Roma tomato, chopped

1 medium-sized red bell pepper, chopped

¼ tsp of ginger, ground

Preparation:

Wash collard greens and lettuce thoroughly under cold running water. Roughly chop it and fill the measuring cups. Reserve the rest for later.

Wash the tomato and place it in a small bowl. Cut into small pieces and reserve the tomato juice while cutting.

Wash the bell pepper and cut lengthwise in half. Remove the seeds and cut into small pieces. Set aside.

Now, combine collard greens, lettuce, tomato, and red bell pepper in a juicer and process until well juiced.

Transfer to a serving glass and stir in the ginger. Add some ice or refrigerate for 10 minutes before serving.

Enjoy!

Nutritional information per serving: Kcal: 61, Protein: 5.5g, Carbs: 17.7g, Fats: 1.1g

35.   Pear Banana Juice

Ingredients:

1 large pear, chopped

1 large banana, sliced

1 cup of pineapple, chunked

1 whole lemon, peeled

5 cherries, pitted

1 tbsp of honey

Preparation:

Wash the pear and cut in half. Remove the core and cut into bite-sized pieces. Set aside.

Peel the banana and cut into small chunks. Set aside.

Cut the top of a pineapple and peel it using a sharp paring knife. Cut into small chunks and fill the measuring cup. Reserve the rest in a refrigerator.

Peel the lemon and cut lengthwise in half. Set aside.

Wash the cherries and cut each in half. Remove the pits and set aside.

Now, combine pear, banana, pineapple, lemon, and cherries in a juicer and process until juiced. Transfer to a serving glass and stir in the honey.

Refrigerate for 10 minutes before serving.

Nutritional information per serving: Kcal: 374, Protein: 4.3g, Carbs: 109g, Fats: 1.2g

36.   Zucchini Avocado Juice

Ingredients:

1 small zucchini, chopped

1 cup of avocado, chunked

1 cup of mango, chopped

1 whole lime, peeled

1 oz coconut water

1 tsp of fresh mint, finely chopped

Preparation:

Peel the zucchini and cut lengthwise in half. Scrape out the seeds and wash it. Cut into small pieces and set aside.

Peel the avocado and cut in half. Remove the pit and cut into chunks. Set aside.

Wash and peel the mango. Chop into bite-sized pieces and set aside.

Peel the lime and cut lengthwise in half. Set aside.

Now, combine zucchini, avocado, mango, lime, and mint in a juicer and process until juiced. Transfer to a serving glass and stir in the coconut water. Add some crushed ice and serve immediately.

Nutritional information per serving: Kcal: 309, Protein: 5.8g, Carbs: 44.5g, Fats: 22.4g

37.   Pumpkin Apricot Juice

Ingredients:

1 cup of pumpkin, chopped

1 cup of apricots, sliced

2 medium-sized strawberries, chopped

1 small Golden Delicious apple, cored

1 tbsp of liquid honey

Preparation:

Peel the pumpkin and cut in half. Scoop out the seeds using a spoon. Cut one large wedge and peel it. Cut into small chunks and fill the measuring cup. Reserve the rest for later.

Wash the apricots and cut each in half. Remove the pits and thinly slice. Set aside.

Wash the strawberries and cut into bite-sized pieces. Set aside.

Wash the apple and remove the core. Cut into small chunks and set aside.

Now, combine pumpkin, apricots, strawberries, and apple in a juicer and process until juiced. Transfer to a serving glass and stir in the honey.

Add some ice and serve.

Nutritional information per serving: Kcal: 222, Protein: 4g, Carbs: 62.3g, Fats: 1.1g

38.   Fennel Artichoke Juice

Ingredients:

1 cup of fennel, chopped

1 medium-sized artichoke, chopped

1 cup of cucumber, sliced

1 medium-sized carrot, sliced

¼ tsp of turmeric, ground

Preparation:

Wash the fennel bulb and trim off the wilted outer layers. Cut into small pieces and fill the measuring cup. Reserve the rest for some other juice.

Trim off the outer leaves of the artichoke using a sharp paring knife. Wash it and cut into bite-sized pieces. Set aside.

Wash and peel the cucumber. Cut into thin slices and fill the measuring cup. Refrigerate the rest for later.

Wash and peel the carrot. Cut into thin slices and set aside.

Now, combine fennel, artichoke, cucumber, and carrot in a juicer a process until well juiced.

Transfer to a serving glass and stir in the turmeric. Add some ice and serve immediately.

Nutritional information per serving: Kcal: 73, Protein: 6.1g, Carbs: 27.5g, Fats: 0.6g

39. Zucchini Tomato Juice

Ingredients:

1 small zucchini, sliced

4 cherry tomatoes, halved

1 medium-sized carrot, sliced

1 small apple, cored

1 whole lime, peeled

Preparation:

Peel the zucchini and cut into thin slices. Set aside.

Wash the cherry tomatoes and cut in half. Set aside.

Wash and peel the carrot. Cut into thin slices and set aside.

Wash the apple and cut lenghtwise in half. Remove the core and cut into bite-sized pieces. Set aside.

Peel the lime and cut lengthwise in half. Set aside.

Now, combine zucchini, tomatoes, carrot, apple, and lime in a juicer and process until well juiced. Transfer to serving glasses and refrigerate before serving.

Nutritional information per serving: Kcal: 119, Protein: 3.4g, Carbs: 35.4g, Fats: 0.9g

40.   Cantaloupe Artichoke Juice

Ingredients:

1 cup of cantaloupe, chopped

1 medium-sized artichoke, chopped

1 medium-sized celery stalk, chopped

1 whole lemon, peeled

1 tbsp of honey

Preparation:

Cut the cantaloupe in half. Scoop out the seeds and cut two wedges and peel them. Chop into chunks and fill the measuring cup. Reserve the rest of the cantaloupe in a refrigerator.

Trim off the outer leaves of the artichoke using a sharp paring knife. Wash it and cut into bite-sized pieces. Set aside.

Wash the celery stalk and cut into bite-sized pieces. Set aside.

Peel the lemon and cut lengthwise in half. Set aside.

Now, combine cantaloupe, artichoke, celery, and lemon in a juicer. Process until juiced. Transfer to a serving glass and stir in the honey.

Add some crushed ice or refrigerate for 15 minutes before serving.

Nutritional information per serving: Kcal: 144, Protein: 6.5g, Carbs: 32.8g, Fats: 0.8g

41.   Pear Cranberry Juice

Ingredients:

2 large pears, chopped

1 cup of cranberries

1 cup of watercress, torn

½ cup of fresh spinach, torn

1 small ginger knob, peeled

Preparation:

Wash the pears and cut in half. Remove the core and cut into bite-sized pieces. Set aside.

Place the cranberries in a colander and rinse thoroughly. Slightly drain and set aside.

Wash watercress and spinach thoroughly under cold running water. Drain and torn with hands. Set aside.

Peel the ginger and set aside.

Now, combine pears, cranberries, watercress, spinach, and ginger in a juicer and process until well juiced. Transfer to a serving glass and stir in some water if you like. However, it is optional.

Refrigerate for 15 minutes before serving.

Enjoy!

Nutritional information per serving: Kcal: 249, Protein: 3.8g, Carbs: 86.1g, Fats: 0.9g

42. Kiwi Guava Juice

Ingredients:

1 whole kiwi, peeled

1 whole guava, peeled

1 cup of mango, chunked

3 whole plums, pitted

1 oz of water

1 tbsp of liquid honey

Preparation:

Peel the kiwi and cut lengthwise in half. Set aside.

Peel the guava and cut into small pieces. Set aside.

Peel the mango and cut into chunks. Set aside.

Wash the plums and cut in half. Remove the pits and cut into bite-sized pieces. Set aside.

Now, combine kiwi, guava, mango, and plums in a juicer. Process until well juiced. Transfer to a serving glass and stir in the water and honey.

Serve cold.

Nutritional information per serving: Kcal: 286, Protein: 4.9g, Carbs: 65.3g, Fats: 2.1g

43.   Pepper Leek Juice

Ingredients:

1 large red bell pepper, chopped

1 whole leek, chopped

1 small zucchini, chopped

1 medium-sized beet, trimmed and chopped

¼ tsp of salt

Preparation:

Wash the bell pepper and cut lengthwise in half. Remove the seeds and cut into small pieces. Set aside.

Wash the leek and cut into bite-sized pieces. Set aside.

Peel the zucchini and cut into bite-sized pieces. Set aside.

Wash the beets and trim off the green ends. peel and cut into small pieces. Set aside.

Now, combine bell pepper, leek, zucchini, and beet in a juicer. Process until juiced. Transfer to a serving glass and stir in the salt.

Refrigerate for 15 minutes before serving.

Enjoy!

Nutritional information per serving: Kcal: 126, Protein: 5.7g, Carbs: 34g, Fats: 1.3g

44.　Sweet Potato Juice

Ingredients:

1 cup of sweet potatoes, chopped

1 cup of asparagus, trimmed

½ cup of green beans, chopped

1 whole lemon, peeled

¼ tsp of turmeric, ground

2 oz of water

Preparation:

Peel the potato and cut into small chunks. Fill the measuring cup and reserve the rest in the refrigerator.

Wash the asparagus and trim off the woody ends. Cut into bite-sized pieces and set aside.

Wash the green beans and cut into small pieces. Set aside.

Peel the lemon and cut lengthwise in half. Set aside.

Now, combine potato, asparagus, green beans, and lemon in a juicer. Process until well juiced. Transfer to a serving glass and stir in the water.

Add some crushed ice and serve immediately.

Nutritional information per serving: Kcal: 135, Protein: 6.1g, Carbs: 39.3g, Fats: 0.5g

45.   Apricot Cauliflower Juice

Ingredients:

2 whole apricots, pitted

1 cauliflower floweret, chopped

1 large carrot, sliced

1 cup of mango, chunked

1 cup of Swiss chard

¼ tsp of ginger, ground

Preparation:

Wash the apricots and cut lengthwise in half. Remove the pits and cut into small pieces. Set aside.

Rinse the cauliflower and roughly chop it. Set aside.

Wash and peel the carrot. Cut into thin slices and set aside.

Wash the mango and cut into small chunks. Fill the measuring cup and reserve the rest for later.

Wash the Swiss chard under cold running water. Slightly drain and roughly chop it. Set aside.

Now, combine apricots, cauliflower, carrot, mango, and Swiss chard in a juicer and process until well juiced.

Transfer to a serving glass and stir in the water and ginger. Add some ice and serve immediately.

Nutritional information per serving: Kcal: 149, Protein: 4.4g, Carbs: 42.5g, Fats: 1.3g

46.   Grapefruit Melon Juice

Ingredients:

1 whole grapefruit, wedged

1 honeydew melon wedge, peeled

1 large banana, sliced

1 whole lime, peeled

1 small orange, wedged

1 tbsp of liquid honey

Preparation:

Peel the grapefruit and divide into wedges. Cut each wedge in half and set aside.

Cut one large honeydew melon wedge and peel it. Remove the seeds and cut into bite-sized pieces. Set aside.

Peel the banana and cut into thin slices. Set aside.

Peel the lime and cut lengthwise in half. Set aside.

Peel the orange and divide into wedges. Cut each wedge in half and set aside.

Now, combine grapefruit, melon, banana, lime, and orange in a juicer and process until juiced.

Transfer to a serving glass and add some ice before serving.

Enjoy!

Nutritional information per serving: Kcal: 281, Protein: 5.2g, Carbs: 83.6g, Fats: 1.2g

47.   Fennel Avocado Juice

Ingredients:

1 cup of fennel, chopped

1 cup of avocado, chunked

1 small Granny Smith's apple, chopped

1 cup of cucumber, sliced

¼ tsp of ginger, ground

Preparation:

Wash the fennel bulb and trim off the wilted outer layers. Cut into small chunks and fill the measuring cup. Reserve the rest in the refrigerator.

Peel the avocado and cut in half. Remove the pit and cut into small chunks. Fill the measuring cup and reserve the rest for later.

Wash the apple and remove the core. Cut into bite-sized pieces and set aside.

Wash the cucumber and cut into thin slices. Fill the measuring cup and reserve the rest in the refrigerator. Set aside.

Now, combine fennel, avocado, apple, and cucumber in a juicer and process until juiced. Transfer to a serving glass and stir in the ginger.

Add some ice before serving.

Nutritional information per serving: Kcal: 286, Protein: 5g, Carbs: 40.3g, Fats: 21.9g

48. Blackberry Banana Juice

Ingredients:

1 cup of blackberries

1 large banana, sliced

1 whole beet, trimmed

1 small green apple, chopped

¼ tsp of cinnamon, ground

Preparation:

Place the blackberries in a colander and rinse well under cold running water. Slightly drain and set aside.

Peel the banana and cut into thin slices. Set aside.

Wash the beet and trim off the green ends. Slightly peel and cut into small pieces. Set aside.

Wash the apple and cut in half. Remove the core and cut into bite-sized pieces. Set aside.

Now, combine blackberries, banana, beet, and apple in a juicer and process until well juiced. Transfer to a serving glass and stir in the cinnamon.

Refrigerate for 15 minutes before serving.

Nutritional information per serving: Kcal: 233, Protein: 5.4g, Carbs: 72.3g, Fats: 1.6g

49. Orange Pomegranate Juice

Ingredients:

1 medium-sized orange, peeled

1 cup of pomegranate seeds

1 small pear, chopped

1 small zucchini, chopped

1 cup of fresh mint, torn

1 tbsp of liquid honey

Preparation:

Peel the orange and divide into wedges. Cut each wedge in half and set aside.

Cut the top of the pomegranate fruit using a sharp paring knife. Slice down to each of the white membranes inside of the fruit. Pop the seeds into a measuring cup and set aside.

Wash the pear and cut in half. Remove the core and cut into bite-sized pieces. Set aside.

Peel the zucchini and cut into small chunks. Set aside.

Rinse the mint under cold running water using a colander. Slightly drain and torn with hands. Set aside.

Now, combine orange, pomegranate seeds, pear, zucchini, and mint in a juicer and process until juiced. Transfer to a serving glass and stir in the honey.

Add some crushed ice and serve immediately.

Nutritional information per serving: Kcal: 259, Protein: 5.6g, Carbs: 61.6g, Fats: 2.1g

50.   Green Sweet Potato Juice

Ingredients:

1 cup of sweet potatoes, chopped

1 cup of turnip greens, torn

1 cup of fresh kale, torn

1 cup of fresh parsley, torn

1 cup of avocado, chunked

1 small green apple, chopped

¼ tsp of ginger, ground

1 tbsp of liquid honey

1 oz of water

Preparation:

Peel the potato and wash it. Cut into small chunks and fill the measuring cup. Reserve the rest in the refrigerator.

Combine turnip greens, kale, and parsley in a large colander. Rinse thoroughly under cold running water. Slightly drain and torn all with hands. Set aside.

Peel the avocado and cut lengthwise in half. Remove the pit and cut into chunks and fill the measuring cup. Reserve the rest for later. Set aside.

Wash the apple and cut in half. Remove the core and cut into bite-sized pieces. Set aside.

Now, combine sweet potato, turnip greens, kale, parsley, avocado, and apple in a juicer and process until juiced. Transfer to a serving glass and stir in the ginger, honey, and water.

Refrigerate for 15 minutes before serving.

Enjoy!

Nutritional information per serving: Kcal: 474, Protein: 11.1g, Carbs: 72.7g, Fats: 23.6g

51. Bean Broccoli Juice

Ingredients:

1 cup of green beans, chopped

1 cup of fresh broccoli, chopped

1 cup of cucumber, sliced

1 cup of mustard greens, torn

1 cup of yam, chopped

1 small ginger knob, peeled

2 oz of water

Preparation:

Wash the green beans and cut into small pieces. Set aside.

Wash the broccoli and cut into bite-sized pieces. Set aside.

Wash the cucumber and cut into thin slices. Fill the measuring cup and reserve the rest for later.

Rinse the mustard greens thoroughly under cold running water. Torn with hands and set aside.

Peel the yam and cut into chunks. Fill the measuring cup and reserve the rest for later.

Peel the ginger knob and set aside.

Now, combine green beans, broccoli, cucumber, mustard greens, yam, and ginger in a juicer and process until juiced.

Transfer to a serving glass and stir in the water.

Add some ice and serve immediately.

Nutritional information per serving: Kcal: 213, Protein: 7.9g, Carbs: 57.2g, Fats: 1.1g

52. Blueberry Cherry Juice

Ingredients:

1 cup of blueberries

1 cup of cherries, pitted

1 cup of black grapes

1 small blood orange, wedged

¼ tsp of cinnamon, ground

Preparation:

Combine blueberries and grapes in a colander and wash under cold running water. Slightly drain and set aside.

Wash the cherries and cut each in half. Remove the pits and set aside.

Peel the orange and divide into wedges. Cut each wedge in half and set aside.

Now, combine blueberries, cherries, grapes, and orange in a juicer and process until juiced.

Transfer to a serving glass and stir in the cinnamon.

Add some ice and serve immediately.

Nutritional information per serving: Kcal: 249, Protein: 4.2g, Carbs: 73.2g, Fats: 1.2g

ADDITIONAL TITLES FROM THIS AUTHOR

70 Effective Meal Recipes to Prevent and Solve Being Overweight: Burn Fat Fast by Using Proper Dieting and Smart Nutrition

By Joe Correa CSN

48 Acne Solving Meal Recipes: The Fast and Natural Path to Fixing Your Acne Problems in Less Than 10 Days!

By Joe Correa CSN

41 Alzheimer's Preventing Meal Recipes: Reduce or Eliminate Your Alzheimer's Condition in 30 Days or Less!

By Joe Correa CSN

70 Effective Breast Cancer Meal Recipes: Prevent and Fight Breast Cancer with Smart Nutrition and Powerful Foods

By Joe Correa CSN